Peppermint Chapstick

2 tbsp. beeswax pastilles

2 tbsp. shea butter

3 tbsp. coconut oil

1 tsp. lanolin (optional)

30+ drops peppermint essential oil (or your scent of choice)

30 empty chapstick tubes

Directions:

Melt beeswax, shea butter and coconut oil in a double boiler or small glass bowl over a small pot of boiling water, stirring constantly until melted.

Remove pan from heat but keep over the still-hot water to keep the mixture melted.

Add essential oils to your preference. Add a few drops at a time and testing a tiny amount on your arm to make sure the scent is to your liking.

Once you've added the essential oils, use the pipette or a dropper to fill the lip balm tubes. This must be done quickly since the mixture will start to harden as soon as it is removed from the heat.

Let tubes sit at room temperature for several hours until cooled and completely hardened before capping them.

Lotion Bars

1 part coconut oil

1 part beeswax

1 part cocoa butter

Essential oil of choice

Directions:

The "1 part" can be whatever you like. 1/2 cup of each, 2 ounces of each, or 1 lb of each. Just use equal parts of each ingredient and you should achieve the right consistency.

Once these three ingredients have been melted over a double boiler, essential oils can be added (if desired). The mixture is then poured into molds and left to harden.

I pour mine into a muffin pan and place into the freezer for 30 minutes (but they can also be left on the counter to cool. They just take a lot longer that way).

Whipped Body Butter

1/3 cup cocoa butter

1/3 cup shea butter

2/3 cup almond oil

1 tsp. Vitamin E oil

15 drops essential oil of choice

Directions:

Combine cocoa butter, shea butter and sweet almond oil into a double boiler, and stir over medium-high heat, until the oils have melted. (If you don't have a double boiler, you can always use a glass bowl set over a pot of boiling water.

Remove from heat, and add Vitamin E oil and essential oil.

Pop into refrigerator for approximately 1 hour. (You want the oils to firm up but not get hard.)

Whip it up with a hand held mixer.

This will last for 6-12 months.

Lightweight Lotion

1 tbsp. grated, tightly packed beeswax

1 tbsp. shea butter

1/2 cup oil (I used sweet almond oil in the recipe pictured above, but olive, apricot kernel, avocado, hazelnut, or another liquid oil will work. Coconut oil is not recommended because it tends to thicken and make the lotion solid.)

2/3 cup water

Directions:

1. Measure your ingredients. Measure twice the amount of water because some will evaporate when it is boiled.

2. Place the water you plan to use as a lotion ingredient in a pot and bring to a boil, then set aside and allow to reach the temperature of hot tea. (Hot, but not so hot that you can't put your pinky in it.)

3. While you're waiting for the water to come to a boil, melt shea butter and beeswax in a separate double boiler. (If you don't have a double boiler you can use a stainless steel bowl set inside a pot of boiling water.) Once the shea butter and beeswax is melted, add the oil and allow to fully melt. Once fully melted, remove the pot from the burner and allow the oils to rest in the double boiler until the water has cooled to the temperature of hot tea described above.

4. Add oil mixture and water to a jar. Place immersion blender at the bottom of the jar and turn it on. Allow it to whir for 15-30 seconds without moving the immersion blender at all. Once the liquid at the bottom is emulsified (which means it has reached a smooth instead of separating like oil and water typically do), begin raising the immersion blender in the liquid to complete the immersion.

5. Once the lotion is fully emulsified, continue to blend every 5-7 minutes until the lotion has cooled to room temperature. Certain oils cool at a different rate than water, which can cause separation if they are not periodically mixed.

Toothpaste

1/2 cup baking soda

1/4 cup extra virgin coconut oil

5 tbsp. xylitol

2 tsp. peppermint extract

Directions:

Combine ingredients and store in a jar or container until ready to use.

Mouthwash

1 16 oz. glass amber jar or mason jar (just store in a dark cabinet) (where to buy)

2 cups distilled or purified water (purified to reduce bacteria and toxins like chlorine and fluoride, can boil on the stove to make distilled water)

1 tsp. xylitol

2 tsp. calcium carbonate powder

5 drops or more of any of the following essential oils – Peppermint, Thieves, Citrus Fresh, Lemon, Orange, Clove and Melaleuca Alternifolia)

Directions:

Boil the container or jar you're going to use for the mouthwash to kill bacteria first.

Put your dry ingredients in the container first.

Add the essential oils to the powders (this will help to disperse the essential oils throughout the solution so they don't just sit on top).

Combine all ingredients in a 16 oz. container (2 cups) and shake well to combine and dissolve.

When using, shake well then pour from the container into a cup so as not to introduce germs to your bottle.

Deoderant

1 tbsp. Coconut Oil

1 tbsp. Cocoa Butter

1 tbsp. Beeswax Pellets

1/2-3/4 tsp. Vitamin E Oil

2 tbsp. Arrowroot Powder or Cornstarch

10 drops Lemongrass Essential Oil or Rosemary Essential Oil

10 drops Tea Tree Essential Oil

Directions:

Combine coconut oil, cocoa butter and beeswax in a small glass bowl.

Place the container in a small saucepan of simmering water to make a fake double boiler. The water should only be half way up the side of your container. Do not get any water into the container.

Watch the mixture carefully and remove from the heat as soon as the beeswax is melted. Use a wooden craft stick or popsicle stick to stir.

Stir in the Vitamin E oil and cornstarch or arrowroot powder until smooth. Remove the sauce pan from the stove but leave the container in the hot water to make the mixing easier. (This keeps the wax hot and melted.)

Once the mixture is smooth stir in your essential oils.

Pour into storage container (you can also use an old deodorant container). Allow the deodorant to cool completely.

Foundation Powder

1/4 cup arrowroot flour starch similar to corn starch (a thickening agent), but without the GMOs.

4 tbsp. unsweetened cocoa powder or cacao powder

1 tsp. ground cinnamon

1/4 tsp. ground nutmeg

1/4 tsp. ground ginger

2 tsp. bentonite clay

10 drops vitamin E oil

12 drops lavender essential oil

Directions:

The amount you use of each ingredient will greatly depend on your skin complexion.

Pour the arrowroot powder in a bowl by itself. Whisk together the cacao powder, cinnamon, ginger, nutmeg and betonite clay in a separate bowl. Slowly add the mixture into the arrowroot powder, testing a small amount on your face (or arm) with your finger or a brush. Keep adding until you get the desired shade of powder.

Blush

2 tbsp. Beet Powder

1 tbsp. Arrowroot Powder

(More or less depending on desired shade)

nutmeg, ground (for darker)

Ginger, ground (for lighter)

Essential oil (I use Lavender)

Directions:

Start with the beet powder as the base. I use around 2 tablespoons of beet powder. Add in the arrowroot powder (I use around 1 tablespoon) depending on how dark or light you desire your blush. Add in a bit of shimmer by adding nutmeg and/or ginger. I usually add nutmeg if I want a darker blush (as pictured) and ginger for a lighter blush. Mix all the dry ingredients until well blended then add in the essential oil (I use 3-5 drops) to give it a bit of "stick". I find this powder wears best when applied with a blush brush.

Eyeliner

2 tsp. coconut oil

4 tsp. aloe vera gel

1 – 2 capsules of activated charcoal (for black) OR ½ tsp cocoa powder (for Brown)

Directions:

Thoroughly mix all ingredients.

Store in an airtight container.

Be sure to store this in a dark and cool place. Use a clean brush to ensure you don't introduce any bacteria to the mixture.

Mascara

1 tsp. coconut oil

1 tsp. shea butter

1 1/2 tsp. beeswax

2 tsp. jojoba oil

2 capsules activated charcoal

2 drops Vitamin E oil

Directions:

In a double boiler, melt the first 4 ingredients

Once melted remove from heat and add in the charcoal and Vitamin E. Cut small corner off plastic bag and use it like a cake decorator to pipe it into the empty mascara tube

Apply your homemade mascara as you would your regular mascara.

Eye Shadows

Arrowroot Powder

Shea Butter

And a combination of any of the following:

Cocoa Powder

Nutmeg

Dried Beet Powder

Turmeric

Allspice

Directions:

1. Start by placing 1/4 – 1/2 tsp. in a small bowl. The more arrowroot powder you use the lighter and more subtle the color of your homemade eyeshadow will be. You can always add more, so start with less.

2. Add your other spices/powders and mix thoroughly until you get the color you desire. (I have four color combinations to get you started below, but have fun and experiment.)

3. Once you have a well-mixed color, add in 1/4 – 1/2 tsp. of shea butter. Use the back of a small spoon to "cream" the butter in with the powder against the side of the bowl until you have a soft, creamy powder. (It really will still look mostly like a powder.) The shea butter will help keep this homemade eyeshadow on your lids and provide a nice moisturizing kick.

Pale Pink:

1/2 tsp. arrowroot powder

1/2 tsp. dried beet powder

1/8 tsp. cocoa powder

1/4 – 1/2 tsp. shea butter

Mauve:

1/2 tsp. arrowroot powder

3/4 tsp. allspice

3/4 tsp. dried beet powder

1/4 tsp. cocoa powder

1/4 – 1/2 tsp. shea butter

Light Brown:

1/2 tsp. arrowroot

3/4 – 1 tsp. cocoa powder

1/4 – 1/2 tsp. shea butter

Golden Brown:

1/2 tsp. arrowroot powder

3/4 tsp. nutmeg

1/4 – 1/2 tsp. turmeric

1/4 – 1/2 tsp. shea butter

Antibiotic Ointment

1/2 cup of coconut oil

1/2 cup of almond oil, grapeseed oil, or olive oil

1/2 cup of the healing herbs of your choice (try chamomile, calendula, comfrey, lavender, plantain leaves etc.

4 tbsp. of beeswax

2 tsp. of witch hazel

15 drops lavender or tea tree essential oils (optional)

Directions:

Put herbs in a glass jar and pour oil over herbs. Make sure they are submerged.

Put glass jar into a saucepan half filled with water. Heat on low heat for 30 minutes. Stir often.

Strain the herbs from the oil with a coffee filter, cheesecloth, t-shirt, etc.

Place strained oil in the jar back into the saucepan with water.

Add the beeswax. Stir well.

Take off the heat once it is fully melted

Add witch hazel and mix

Once cooled, put into a container of choice and store in a cool, dark place. (Keeps for up to a year.)

Apply directly to scrapes, cuts, burns, diaper rash, dry skin, athlete's foot, etc. as required.

Burn & Sunburn Ointment

1/4 cup raw honey, preferably Manuka honey 1/4 cup unrefined coconut oil

1 tsp. beeswax

1 tbsp. Sea Buckthorn oil, optional

1/2 tsp. aloe vera gel, aloe vera juice, or rosewater

Directions:

In a small, heavy-bottomed saucepan or double boiler, heat the beeswax over the lowest heat possible.

When the beeswax is nearly melted, add in the coconut oil and melt completely.

Stir in the honey and Sea Buckthorn oil, if using, and whisk over the heat only until the whole mixture is one uniform liquid, about 30 seconds.

Remove from the heat and either pour directly into tins or other containers OR stir in the aloe or rosewater briskly until the mixture is completely homogenous, then pour into your containers.

Let sit until comfortable to touch before using. The mixture will fully harden in approximately 6-12 hours.

Homemade Antibiotic

1 garlic clove

2 tbsp. honey

2 tbsp. ginger powder

1/2 tbsp. ground chili peppers

1/2 tbsp. cinnamon

3.3 oz fresh lemon juice

Directions:

Crush garlic and set aside for 10-15 minutes. This activates it's most powerful compound, allicin.

Add crushed garlic, ginger powder, chili powder and cinnamon to the lemon juice.

Mix these ingredients.

Stir in the honey.

Let the syrup rest for 3 hours on a room temperature. Keep the syrup in a glass jar with a lid and store it in the fridge.

How To Use: Take 1 tablespoon daily to strengthen your immune system. If you're suffering from an infection, take 1 tablespoon of the syrup, three times a day before each meal.

What Each Ingredient Does

1. Garlic

Garlic is both an antibiotic and an antiseptic, meaning that is capable of preventing infection by inhibiting the growth of infectious agents as well as treating an infection as it occurs. It even works against bacteria resistant to penicillin and amoxicillin.

2. Honey

Honey is an antimicrobial agent that can be applied topically for prevention or treatment of infections, including those caused by multi drug-resistant bacteria.

It fights bacteria by acidity, osmotic effect, high sugar concentration and polyphenols and by producing hydrogen peroxide. These different methods make it harder for bacteria to develop resistance.

While these different method are highly effective in killing bacteria, they do not damage healthy cells.

3. Ginger

Ginger has been shown to have an antibacterial effect on respiratory and periodontal infections. Ginger can also fight drug–resistant fungi.

4. Chili Peppers

Unlike some natural remedies which rely on one specific genus of a spice, like cinnamon, 4 different varieties of chili pepper have antibiotic effects. They have been used in Mayan medicine for thousands of years.

In fact, Capsicum baccatum, Capsicum chinese, Capsicum frutescens, and Capsicum pubescens varieties were found to have antimicrobial effects against fifteen bacterial species and one yeast species.

These peppers contain two different antibiotic compounds capsaicin and dihydrocapsaicin.

5. Cinnamon

A study lead by a team of surgeons, for example, found that a solution made with cinnamon oil killed a number of common and hospital-acquired infections, like streptococcus and methicillin-resistant Staphylococcus aureus, or MRSA.

6. Lemon

Citric acid from lemon juice has proven to prevent the highly contagious norovirus from infecting humans. It's considered to be a safe disinfectant to be used in the home and kitchen.

Lemon essential oil is a mild antibacterial, antiviral, antifungal and anti-inflammatory, For stronger benefits, include lemon peel in the remedy

Cough Syrup

2 cups water

8 sprigs fresh thyme

¼ cup fresh ginger root, finely chopped

1 cup raw honey

1 lemon, juiced

⅛ tsp. cayenne pepper

Directions:

Put water, thyme, and chopped ginger into a pot.

Simmer the herbs in water until reduced by half.

Allow to cool until the temperature is warm, not hot, steeping the herbs the entire time.

Strain. Discard or compost the thyme and ginger.

Return the thyme-ginger tea to the pot.

Whisk in honey, lemon juice, and cayenne pepper.

Transfer to an airtight jar or bottle.

Syrup will keep in a dark cupboard for 1 week. After that, it should be stored in the refrigerator.

Administer a tablespoon as often as necessary to soothe a sore throat and calm a cough.

Chest Cold Remedy Bars

4 oz. Coconut Oil

4 oz. Raw Shea Butter

4 oz. Beeswax Pellets

Essential Oils - Eucalyptus, Peppermint &

Rosemary

Silicone Mold

Double Boiler

Directions:

melt together the shea butter, coconut oil, and beeswax, stirring frequently. Mix in 15 drops of peppermint oil, 10 drops of Eucalyptus oil, and 10 drops of rosemary oil.

Carefully pour the liquid into the silicone mold and allow to sit undisturbed until completely cool and firm (approximately 60-90 minutes depending on temperature and humidity). Once the chest rub bars are cool, it's easy to pop them out of the mold.

The bars are solid at room temperature, but once you begin to rub the bar onto your skin, the body heat will melt it enough to leave behind a thin layer of moisturizing lotion and essential oils that will help battle your cough and cold symptoms. Rub the bar on your chest (and/or the bottoms of your feet) at bedtime every night.

Cough Drops

½ cup of raw honey

2 tbsp. lemon juice

1 tsp. freshly grated ginger root

few drops of peppermint oil

Kitchen items you will need: a candy thermometer, a candy mold with small openings. You can make the cough drops without the mold; oil a piece of parchment paper and pour the candy onto it. Let it harden, and then break it up into small pieces.

Directions:

Measure the honey, lemon juice, and grated ginger and pour it all into a saucepan.

With a wire whisk, stir the mixture as it heats to a boil. It will become foamy and start to climb up the sides of the pan, remove it from the heat and continue to whisk it until the foam reduces and then put it back over the heat. Repeat this until a candy thermometer reads 300 degrees, you will want to check frequently because the honey heats fast and scorches easily!

Drop a bit of the mixture into a glass of ice water (or, dip a spoon into the mixture and then quickly dip it into the ice water). If the mixture forms a hard, crunchy ball, it's ready! If not, keep up with the whisking and heating and try again in a minute or so. Once a hard ball forms in the ice water, you're good to go!

Let the mixture cool until the foam has reduced. Then, very carefully, drizzle the candy into the mold (or onto the oiled parchment paper). Let it cool in a safe place (not the freezer or fridge) until the cough drops are hard. When they are hard, press on the back of the mold to release. Or, if you're not using a mold, break the cough drops up into pieces.

Store in an airtight container. These actually do better in the fridge, as they attract moisture and tend to get sticky if left out.

Hair Conditioner

2 to 4 tbsp. raw shea butter

½ to 1 cup of coconut milk

2 tsp. raw honey

3 to 5 drops of desired essential oil

Directions:

Into your food processor, add raw shea butter, coconut milk and honey. Blend for 10 seconds or more, depending on your blender, until you get a thick liquid.

And your shea butter hair conditioner is ready! Now all you need to do is transfer it to a glass jar. It's not a leave-in conditioner so make sure to rinse it out after.

Then add 3 to 5 drops of any essential oil. Shake well to combine. You can store it in the refrigerator for up to a week or more.

Headache Salve

2 tbsp. dried mint leaves, crumbled

2 tbsp. dried pine needles, chopped

⅔ cup sunflower or olive oil

1 tbsp. tamanu oil

½ oz. beeswax

½ t. - ¾ tsp. peppermint essential oil

Directions:

Infuse the mint leaves and pine needles into the sunflower or olive oil. Once it has sufficiently infused, strain the oil. You can store this infused oil for up to 9-12 months before making the salve. When you're ready to make the salve, combine ½ cup of the infused oil with the tamanu and beeswax in a canning jar or other heatproof container. Set the container down into a small saucepan containing 1-2" of water, then place the pan over a medium-low burner until the beeswax has melted.

Remove from heat and stir in the peppermint oil. Carefully pour the hot mixture into tins or jars.

Depending on your preference, you may want a softer or firmer salve. If so, just remelt the product and add a pinch more beeswax for a firmer consistency or a little more oil for a softer salve. Shelf life of the salve is around 6-9 months, if stored in a cool location, out of direct sunlight.

Cold Process Soap (Bars)

14 oz. sodium hydroxide (Lye)

2.28 lbs. of distilled water

2.5 lbs. of Olive Oil

1.5 lbs. of Coconut Oil (76 degree)

0.5 lb. of Sweet Almond Oil

1.5 lbs. of Palm Oil or Palm Kernel Flakes

3 oz. of Fragrance

Directions:

Weigh, do not measure, your oils on a home kitchen scale. Don't spend the extra money on extra virgin. Even oxidized oils are fine for soap. Mix all the melted oils together into a bucket.

Weigh, do not measure, your sodium hydroxide into a plastic container. Weigh or measure your distilled water into the second large bucket. Measured and weighed ounces of water are the same, but the math can get you.

Carefully, and slowly, OUTSIDE, pour the sodium hydroxide into the water, being careful not to get any splashes on you. WARNING! DON'T BREATH THE FUMES. HOLD YOUR BREATH WHILE YOU POUR AND BRIEFLY STIR THE

CONTENTS WITH YOUR LONG SPOON TO DISSOLVE THE GRANULES. THE MIXTURE WILL BE HOT.

Wait for the mixture to cool to 100 degrees F.

Pour the sodium hydroxide water into the bucket of oils, stirring as you go. Be careful not to get any on you. It is still very caustic at this point. Don't be afraid of the warnings. Follow them and you'll be fine. Just be aware that even after mixing we are dealing with nasty stuff here.

Mix the soap until it "traces," meaning that when you take some in the spoon and drizzle it back, it takes a second for the ripple to go down. It means that you have mixed it enough and the chemical reaction is taking place. Time to trace can be 15 minutes or an hour. Just keep stirring periodically at the very least, and make sure you get down into the corners of the bucket. You can use an electric beater mixer, but you need a tray type of bucket so that the beaters reach the bottom. Use low speed.

Add your fragrance as a last step and mix it in good. Some essential oils can speed up a trace quite a bit so beware that you might have to get moving.

Pour the soap from the bucket into the lined mold.

Cover the entire mold with a blanket for 24-48 hours.

When it seems to have solidified you can cut the mold away or take apart your purchased molds.

One week later you can cut the soap. Don't worry about perfectly shaped bars unless you decide to buy a cutter system. A guitar string works great.

When you cut the soap, lay it out on racks to dry. They don't have to be actual metal racks. Cardboard works fine and the bars don't stick.

In about 6 weeks the bars will be totally cured. You can use one before then but it will feel slippery because of the alkaline PH.

Castile Liquid Soap

32 1/8 oz. Coconut oil

48 oz. Olive oil

32 oz. (4 cups | 907 grams) distilled water

9.35 oz. weight (265 grams) Potassium hydroxide lye flakes

10 cups Distilled water (For diluting after)

Directions:

Measure out the coconut and olive oil and begin to heat it over low heat. I warmed mine on the low setting of my slow cooker. A slow cooker is perfect for this sort of job because it will gently warm without burning, and keeping things at a steady temperature.

Measure out the potassium hydroxide (KOH).

Carefully add the KOH to the water (and not the other way around!) in a well ventilated area. I usually do this outside. Stir the KOH into the water until it dissolves. It will be cloudy at first, but then it will clear up.

Slowly add in the the KOH mixture to the warm oils, and slowly stir them together in the slow cooker over low heat to incorporate the lye mixture into the oils.

Using a hand held blender, begin to blend the ingredients together in the slow cooker. In a few minutes the mixture will begin to thicken and look like mayonnaise, and then just moments later will look like a creamy pudding.

A couple of minutes later, the mixture will begin to look grainy. A lot of people call this the mashed potatoes stage because that's sort of what the mixture resembles. Continue to blend. (If at any point the mixture becomes too thick to blend with the hand held blender, switch to mixing with a wooden spoon.

As you continue to blend, it will start to get creamy again, and you will notice that you will start to see translucent streaks in your mixture. Once you reach this point, you can stop blending with the hand held blender, and begin to stir occasionally with a wooden spoon.

The mixture will begin to thicken up and become more translucent. We are now working on making a soap base paste which will be dissolved into a clear liquid soap. The process will take 3-4 hours, and you will want to check on it and stir it up every half an hour or so.

To check for "doneness," we will look to see if our paste is dissolving into a completely clear liquid soap. To do this, take a small amount of the soap paste and dissolve it in water, and look to see if the water is clear once the soap paste is dissolved. If the liquid is cloudy, you will want to continue to cook the soap in the slow cooker. You can let it cook another half an hour before checking on it again. If it dissolves clear like the soap in my picture, you are finished making the soap paste.

Your liquid castile soap paste is now ready to be stored or dissolved into liquid soap as needed.

Diluting Your Soap Paste

Once the soap paste has fully gelled, proceed with dilution. Like the cook phase, dilution of the paste is a slow process, but the soap will pretty much take care of itself.

Add 10 cups distilled water to the soap paste in the crockpot. Break up the soap paste into the water into smaller blobs of paste as best you can but don't worry about the paste dissolving yet.

Turn the crock pot heat to keep-warm, lid the crockpot and give the soap paste all day or overnight to dissolve. If possible, every hour, or as you happen to think of it, give the soap a stir to help it along.

If, after 8 hours-ish, you're still seeing a lot of chunks of soap, or you see a skin forming at the top of the soap, add in another cup of distilled water and let the soap continue to dissolve. Repeat with the final cup of distilled water if needed.

When your soap is fully dissolved with no chunks of soap paste remaining, it's ready to bottle.

Baby Wipes

1 1/4 - 1 1/2 cups distilled water (or boiled and cooled)

1 tbsp. castile soap

1 tbsp. aloe vera gel

1 tbsp. witch hazel

1/2 tbsp. oil (olive, sweet almond, or coconut)

10-15 drops essential oils

1 roll strong paper towels (Bounty or Viva)

Storage container (old wipes container, or tupperware)

Directions:

Cut the roll of paper towels in half with a sharp, non-serrated knife.

Place one half of the roll in a tall container (or accordion fold the towels and place in an old wipes container).

In a small bowl, add the water, castile soap, aloe vera, witch hazel, and almond oil, and stir to mix well.

Add the essential oils and stir to combine.

Slowly pour mixture over the towels to saturate them. If you're using a wipes container, just pull the towels through the little slot in the cover and you're done!

If using a tall container, flip it over after 5-10 minutes to make sure the towels are completely wet with the solution. Then flip it back over, pull out the cardboard roll from the middle and the first towel should come right out.

Use as you would regular baby wipes.

1. This recipe is for one half of the paper towel roll. Depending on the brand and size of your towels, you may need to adjust the amounts of water and soap in the recipe.

2. If using reusable cloth wipes, just pour the solution into a shallow pan and place the cloth wipes in the solution until they're saturated. Then just place the wipes into an old wipes container and use as you would regular wipes.

Lavendar, Rosemary Shampoo

1/2 cup Castile Soap

1 1/2 cups distilled water

3 tsp. virgin coconut oil

1 – 3 drops Lavender essential oil

1 – 3 drops Rosemary essential oil

Directions:

Melt coconut oil in a microwave safe dish. It should only take about 20-30 seconds to become fully liquefied.

Combine water, coconut oil , castile soap, and essential oils in a pint mason jar and shake vigorously to combine.

Pour into a plastic container to store and use. An empty shampoo bottle is a great container or you can pick up a new pump or squeeze bottle.

How to use homemade shampoo:

Squirt a quarter sized amount of shampoo into the palm of your hand.

Rub hands together to create lather.

Massage shampoo through hair, beginning at the roots.

Rinse hair well with water as cold as you can tolerate; the cold water will seal your ends and provide a greater shine.

Coconut Milk & Honey Shampoo

1/2 cup liquid castille soap

1/4 cup honey

1/4 cup coconut milk

2 tbsp. jojoba oil

1 tbsp. vitamin E oil (optional)

30-40 drops essential oils

Directions:

Combine all ingredients in a re-purposed shampoo bottle, or a soap dispenser. Old dressing bottles also work. Shake before each use, (because, as you can tell, it will separate) and use as

you would regular shampoo.